This book is intended for informational purposes only. It is not a substitute for professional medical advice, diagnosis, or treatment. Always seek the advice of your physician or other qualified healthcare provider with any questions you may have regarding a medical condition.

Published in the United States of America.

For permissions, inquiries, or additional resources, please visit: www.eatthetrees.com

"Let the leaves be for the healing of the nations." – Revelation 22:2.

Table of Contents

Table of Contents (Continued)

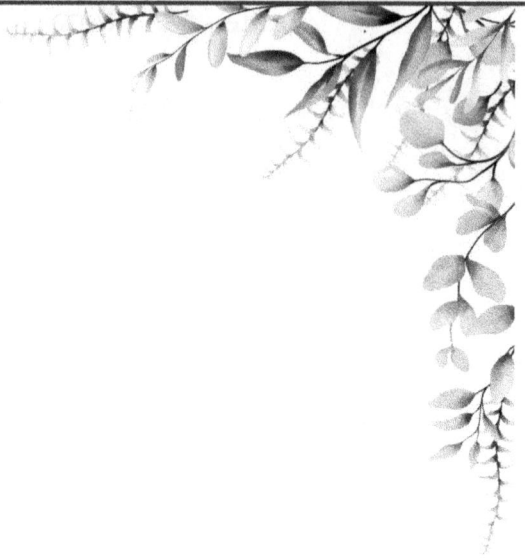

This book is lovingly dedicated to my family; too many to name but too dear to my heart to forget.

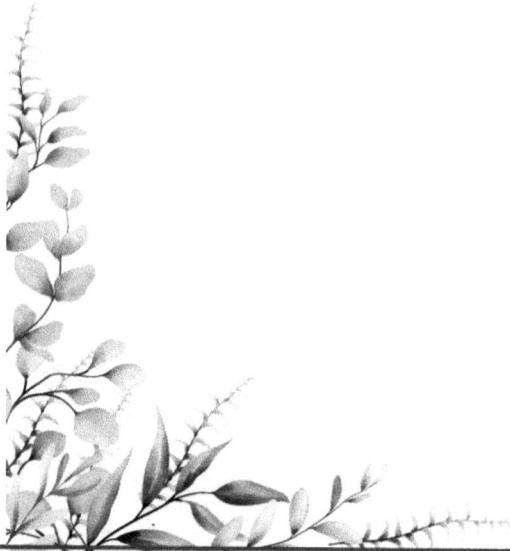

Disclaimer

The information presented in this book is for educational and informational purposes only and is not intended as medical advice. I am a Certified Autoimmune Holistic Nutrition Specialist and Vegan Transition Coach—not a licensed physician. Always consult your doctor or healthcare provider before making any changes to your diet, lifestyle, or supplement routine, especially if you are managing a chronic condition or are on medication.

This book is based on personal experience, professional training, and spiritual study. It is not intended to diagnose, treat, cure, or prevent any disease.

Please understand that each person is bio-individual—what works well for one may not work the same way for another. Listen to your body, track your progress, and make choices that support your unique path to healing.

This book may also reference spiritual practices such as prayer, meditation, and energy alignment. These practices are shared from a place of personal conviction and should be engaged with according to your own beliefs and comfort level.

By reading this book, you acknowledge full responsibility for your own health choices and outcomes.

Welcome to your healing.

If you've picked up this book, chances are...
you're tired.

Tired of chronic symptoms, tired of prescriptions
that mask rather than mend, tired of trying to
feel better but not knowing where to begin.

I see you. I am you. And I created this book to
help you stop surviving and start nourishing —
not with another overwhelming diet plan or rigid
food rules, but with a return to the wisdom of
plants.

The pages ahead are rooted in holistic, plant-
powered healing, designed to support chronic
conditions like diabetes, inflammation,
autoimmune disorders, fatigue, and more — all
from the lens of love, simplicity, and restoration.

Inside, you'll find:

- Clear explanations of root causes (not just
  symptoms)
- Nutrient-dense foods that help the body heal
- Simple recipes and supplement suggestion
- Encouragement to eat mindfully and speak
  life over your meals; and

- Spiritual nourishment — because we are body, mind, and spirit

I call this "eating the trees and drinking the leaves" — a sacred way of healing that's been gifted to us from the beginning of time. The food is already here. It's time to let it do its work.

You don't have to be perfect. You don't have to do it all at once.

You just have to begin — one meal at a time.

Let's walk this healing path together.

With love,
Patty Johnson Militello

The Truth in Numbers: Chronic Illness and the Call for Change

Chronic diseases are the leading cause of death and disability in the United States, and the burden is especially heavy on women—particularly women of color.

- 6 in 10 adults in the U.S. live with at least one chronic disease; 4 in 10 have two or more.
- Autoimmune diseases affect approximately 80% women—with many women remaining undiagnosed for years. Black and Latina women face even greater delays in diagnosis and care.
- 1 in 10 women over age 20 lives with type 2 diabetes—and many more are in the prediabetic stage without knowing it.
- Stroke is the third leading cause of death in women, with women more likely than men to suffer long-term disability.
- Black women are more likely to be prescribed medication and less likely to be offered lifestyle interventions, despite

research showing that food, movement, and stress management play a powerful role in healing.

These numbers are not just statistics—they are stories, mothers, daughters, sisters, aunties, and grandmothers. They are the reason Eat the Trees, Drink the Leaves exists: to empower women with knowledge, nourish them with whole, healing foods, and remind them that radiant health is their birthright.

How to Use This Book

This guide was created to support you — whether you're managing a chronic condition or simply seeking a plant-powered lifestyle that brings your body back into balance.

Each section focuses on a specific area of healing, such as blood sugar balance, inflammation, or stroke recovery. You do not need to read it in order. Instead, use the section(s) that speak most to your needs right now.

Every chapter includes these elements to guide your healing:

- **Root Causes** – A simple explanation of what's happening in your body and why.
- **Key Nutrients** – The most important vitamins, minerals, and compounds that help restore balance.
- **Healing Foods** – Everyday plant-based foods that provide what your body needs to recover.
- **Sample Recipe** – A nourishing meal idea to try (easy and flexible!).
- **Supplement Suggestions** – Natural supports to consider (with a reminder to consult your doctor

- **Coach's Corner** – Words of encouragement, wisdom, and real talk — just for you.

You'll also find tools like my Nourishment Tracker, a Spiritual Support page with affirmations and scriptures to help align your body and spirit, and for a small price ($7), you can obtain my Glow Deeper: Build-Your-Own Healing Bowl Matrix.

Above all, let this book serve as a "gentle companion." There's no pressure to do it all. Healing is not a race — it's a return. A return to wholeness.

Honoring Your Bio-Individuality

Because your healing path is sacred and unique...

No two bodies are alike—and neither are their healing journeys. In this guide, you'll find nourishing tools, plant-powered recipes, and heartfelt reflections rooted in holistic wisdom. But always remember this: what supports one woman's healing may not support yours in the same way. That's the beauty of bio-individuality.

Your genes, environment, medical history, culture, energy, and spiritual walk all contribute to what your body needs in this moment. And those needs will shift and evolve as you grow.

Maybe raw greens give you energy, or maybe they leave you bloated. Maybe turmeric feels like medicine to your soul, or maybe your body prefers ginger's warmth. There is no shame, only wisdom, in honoring your truth.

This journey invites you to:
- Listen deeply to your body's cues and rhythms
- Release the pressure to follow what works for others
- Embrace your story with grace, curiosity, and gentleness; and
- Adapt each suggestion, meal, or supplement to what aligns with you.

You don't have to follow this plan perfectly. You don't need to adopt every single suggestion. You're allowed to pause. You're allowed to pivot.

Take what nourishes you and leave the rest. This is your path, your body, your healing. With every bite, breath, and intention—you're choosing renewal. That's the most powerful medicine of all.

Pantry Detox & Clean Eating Guide

Your kitchen is your sanctuary—a sacred space where healing begins. Before diving into recipes or stocking up on healing foods, it's time for a pantry refresh. Removing foods that hinder your body's natural healing process is the first act of self-love in this journey.

Step 1: Remove These Common Triggers

Clear your pantry and fridge of items that promote inflammation, blood sugar spikes, or digestive distress:

- Processed snacks (chips, crackers, packaged baked goods)
- Refined sugar and artificial sweeteners (high-fructose corn syrup, aspartame)
- White flour and processed grains
- Dairy products (cheese, milk, cream)
- Conventional meats (especially cured, deli, or factory-farmed)
- Canola, soybean, and vegetable oils
- Artificial colors and preservatives

Tip: Don't toss everything—donate unopened items or share with others who may still use them.

Step 2: Restock with Healing Staples

Now it's time to restock with foods that nourish, energize, and support your healing:

- Whole Grains: Quinoa, brown rice, millet, oats
- Legumes: Lentils, chickpeas, black beans
- Nuts & Seeds: Walnuts, chia seeds, flaxseeds, hemp hearts
- Plant-Based Oils: Olive oil, avocado oil, coconut oil (sparingly)
- Herbs & Spices: Turmeric, ginger, garlic, cinnamon, cayenne, rosemary
- Sweeteners: Dates, coconut sugar, pure maple syrup (in moderation)
- Non-Dairy Milks: Unsweetened almond, oat, or coconut milk
- Fresh & Frozen Produce: Focus on variety, color, and seasonal availability
- Fermented Foods: Sauerkraut, kimchi, coconut yogurt, kombucha

Step 3: Mindful Meal Prep Tools

Support your new lifestyle with helpful tools:

- Glass food storage containers
- Blender or food processor
- Steamer basket or air fryer
- Mason jars for teas and smoothies
- A good chef's knife and cutting board

Building a Healing Bowl: The ROOTS Method

Welcome to the heart of this journey — The ROOTS Method™. **This simple, powerful framework helps you build a healing bowl that feeds not just your body, but your spirit and sense of purpose.**

ROOTS stands for:

- **R**ooted in Nature
- **O**rganic & Whole
- **O**verflowing with Nutrients
- **T**herapeutic by Design
- **S**acred Self-Care

Each bowl is a celebration of plant wisdom, ancestral healing, and your personal path to wholeness. Whether you're just starting out or deep in your wellness journey, the ROOTS Method helps you create meals that are healing, balanced, and deeply satisfying.

How to Build a Healing Bowl Using the ROOTS Method

1. **Start with a Base (R – Rooted in Nature)**
- Think leafy greens, ancient grains, sea vegetables, or hearty cruciferous veggies. These are your grounding foods.

2. **Add Colorful Variety (O – Organic & Whole)**
- Use organic, seasonal produce—rainbow carrots, roasted beets, purple cabbage, golden squash. Let your bowl look like a garden in bloom.

3. **Boost with Nutrients (O – Overflowing with Nutrients)**
- Sprinkle in nuts, seeds, fermented foods, or mineral-rich herbs. Add omega-3s, B-vitamins, and iron-rich greens.

4. **Include Healing Components (T – Therapeutic by Design)**
- Turmeric, ginger, garlic, miso, or medicinal mushrooms—use intentional ingredients that support your condition or goals.

5. **Finish with Love (S – Sacred Self-Care)**
- Drizzle a homemade dressing. Add a prayer or intention. Eat slowly and give thanks for the healing and the nourishment.

My Healing Journey: A Personal Encounter with a Stroke

It was a Friday afternoon when I was getting ready to leave work. I was looking forward to the weekend. No big plans, just happy for the break; but something felt off. Out of nowhere, I felt a buzz, a vibration near the top of my head. My body weakened like I was living in slow motion. My words began to slur. Something definitely wasn't right. That moment—unexpected and terrifying—was the beginning of a life-altering chapter.

In that instant life tilted beneath my feet. Time slowed, the noise of my world dissolved, and every plan—big or small, important or routine—slipped away like mist. The errands I meant to run, the meals I had yet to cook, even the thoughts circling in my mind... all of it vanished in a single heartbeat. What remained was my body on the floor crying out in distress and my spirit stretching toward meaning, clinging to the fragile hope that I would make it through whatever this was.

The faces of my children rose in my mind, and tears welled in my eyes before I could stop them. In that fragile space between fear and hope, I whispered a thousand prayers—pleading for grace to see them again.

I asked forgiveness for every wrong, spoken or unspoken, and begged for mercy to fulfill my purpose if it was not yet complete.

Oh, but God...

With divine grace, wisdom, and spiritual guidance, I turned inward and upward. I knew this was a wake-up call—not just for me, but for every woman I may have the opportunity to serve. I began applying every healing tool I ever shared with others: anti-inflammatory foods, healing teas, deep rest, prayer, meditation, and forgiveness, and I researched, studied, and applied new tools.

I was released from one hospital a week and a half after the stroke with no walking cane nor any other assistance. I passed every cognitive test given to me. My release from physical and occupational therapy was just over a month later.

I gave my body the permission it longed for—to rest, to mend, to heal. I opened the door of my heart and allowed it to feel fully, without restraint. And to my soul, I offered freedom—the gentle invitation to shine, to glow, to radiate life once more.

Today, I don't just teach healing—I embody it.

My hope is that this section meets you exactly where you are. Whether you are healing from a stroke, supporting someone who is, or learning how to prevent one—please know this: your life still has divine purpose, and your healing can begin today.

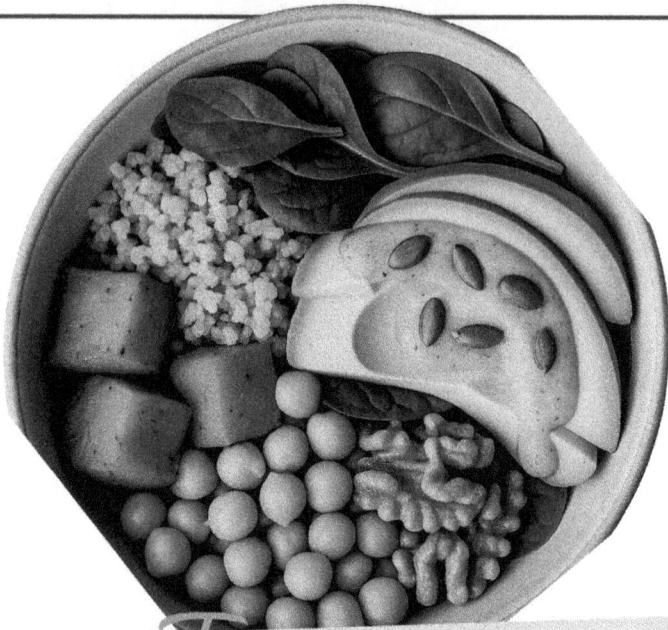

Focus on

STROKES

"Stroke Recovery: Rising from the Storm"

When life shifts in an instant, so does the path beneath your feet. A hemorrhagic stroke may have altered your rhythm, but it didn't cancel your calling.

Recovery is not just about regaining function—it's about rediscovering your purpose, rebuilding trust in your body's ability to heal, and recognizing the miracle of every breath.

A stroke occurs when blood flow to the brain is disrupted, depriving brain cells of oxygen and essential nutrients. This interruption can result from a clot blocking an artery (ischemic stroke) or a blood vessel bursting (hemorrhagic stroke).

ROOT CAUSES

Strokes can stem from a combination of root causes, including:

- **High blood pressure (the leading contributor)**
- **Plaque buildup and atherosclerosis**
- **High blood sugar and insulin resistance**
- **Chronic inflammation and oxidative stress**
- **Lack of physical activity and nutrient deficiency**

Healing begins by restoring balance through plant-based foods that reduce inflammation, support vascular health, and nourish the brain's recovery process.

KEY NUTRIENTS

- **Magnesium** – Supports nerve repair and blood pressure regulation
- **Omega-3 fatty acids** – Reduce inflammation and promote brain cell communicat

- **Vitamin B12 & Folate** – Essential for nerve health and cognitive support
- **CoQ10** – Supports energy production in cells, particularly in the heart and brain
- **Vitamin D3 + K2** – Aids vascular health and reduces arterial calcification
- **Turmeric (Curcumin)** – A powerful anti-inflammatory to support post-stroke recovery

HEALING FOODS

- Leafy greens (kale, spinach, Swiss chard)
- Berries (antioxidant-rich for brain health)
- Walnuts, chia, and flaxseeds (plant-based omega-3s)
- Avocados (healthy fats and potassium)
- Garlic and turmeric (circulation and inflammation support)
- Beets (natural nitric oxide boost for blood flow)
- Lentils and black beans (fiber + folate combo)

RECIPES

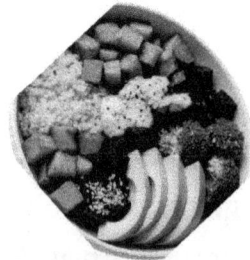

BRAIN BOOSTING BOWL

A colorful, healing dish designed to support cognitive clarity, reduce inflammation, and help restore energy after a stroke or chronic fatigue.

Ingredients (Serves 2)

For the Bowl:
- 1 cup cooked quinoa (½ cup dry)
- 1 small beet, peeled and chopped into small cubes
- 1 small, sweet potato, peeled and chopped into small cubes
- 1 cup broccoli florets
- 1 ripe avocado, sliced
- 2 tablespoons hemp seeds

For the Tahini-Lemon Dressing:
- 2 tablespoons tahini
- 1 tablespoon fresh lemon juice
- 1 teaspoon maple syrup (optional)

Optional Boosts:
- Add a handful of baby spinach for extra greens
- Sprinkle with pumpkin seeds or walnut pieces for crunch
- Serve with a side of lemon water or a calming tea for digestion

BLUEBERRY BRAIN-BOOST SMOOTHIE

Ingredients:
- 1 cup unsweetened almond milk (or any non-dairy milk)
- ½ cup frozen blueberries
- ½ frozen banana
- ¼ avocado (for healthy fats)
- 1 tbsp ground flaxseed or chia seeds
- 1 tsp hemp seeds
- 1 tsp raw honey or date syrup (optional)
- ½ tsp ground cinnamon
- ½ tsp turmeric (anti-inflammatory)
- ½ tsp vanilla extract
- 3–4 ice cubes (optional)

Instructions:
1. Add all ingredients to a high-speed blender.
2. Blend until smooth and creamy.
3. Pour into a glass, sprinkle with a pinch of cinnamon or hemp seeds on top and enjoy.

Benefits: *This smoothie is rich in brain-protective antioxidants, omega-3s, fiber, and anti-inflammatory compounds to support cognitive function and blood flow.*

STROKE SUPPORT HERBAL SIPPING TEA

Ingredients:
- 1 tsp dried hibiscus petals
- 1 tsp dried lemon balm
- 1 tsp dried rosemary
- ½ tsp grated fresh ginger (or ¼ tsp ground)
- 1 small strip of orange peel (optional)
- 2 cups hot water
- Raw honey or stevia (optional)

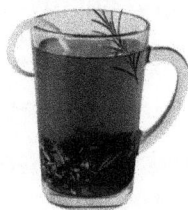

Instructions:
1. Combine all herbs in a teapot or infuser.
2. Pour hot water over herbs and steep for 8–10 minutes.
3. Strain into your favorite mug and sweeten if desired.
4. Sip slowly while resting or journaling.

Benefits: *Hibiscus and rosemary support circulation and blood pressure, lemon balm calms the nervous system, and ginger enhances blood flow—all gentle allies for stroke recovery.*

SUPPLEMENT SUGGESTIONS

> Always consult your healthcare provider before starting new supplements, especially if you're on medications or have a medical condition.

These supplements support brain healing, circulation, and nervous system recovery:

1. **Omega-3 Fatty Acids (EPA/DHA)** - Supports brain cell repair, reduces inflammation, and promotes circulation.
2. **Curcumin (from Turmeric)** - Natural anti-inflammatory that may support brain health and reduce oxidative stress.
3. **Vitamin D3 with K2** - Helps reduce inflammation and supports vascular and immune health. K2 ensures calcium is used correctly.
4. **Magnesium Glycinate** - Calms the nervous system, supports brain and muscle recovery, and reduces cramping or spasms.
5. **N-Acetyl Cysteine (NAC)** - Boosts glutathione production to protect the brain from oxidative damage.
6. **CoQ10** - Supports mitochondrial energy and cardiovascular recovery.
7. **Ginkgo Biloba** - Improves circulation to the brain and may enhance memory and cognitive recovery.

8. **B-Complex (with B6, B9, and B12)** - Supports nerve repair and reduces homocysteine levels, which can protect against future stroke risk.

COACH'S CORNER

Dear Sister, this moment is sacred. Whether you are on your own healing journey or walking beside someone you love, please know that healing is not only possible—it is within reach.

1. Start gently.
Your body has been through a storm. Now is the time to rebuild, one nourishing bite, one breath of grace at a time. Begin each day with hydration and grounding foods. Blend in anti-inflammatory herbs, gentle movement, and rest.

2. Remember:
Your plate is your power. Each forkful of healing greens, each sip of mineral-rich tea is a quiet protest against disease and a bold declaration of life.

3. Lean into love and connection.
Whether you're celebrating a small win or navigating a difficult day, know that love, community, and faith will carry you farther than you can imagine.

4. Prioritize spiritual wellness.
Prayer, meditation, quiet reflection, and nature walks are not extras—they are essentials. They help calm your nervous system and restore your heart.

5. You are the testimony.
Your story will bless others. Never forget that your body is sacred, your healing is holy, and your journey is valid—no matter how slow or winding the path may be.

7-Day Healing Wellness Tracker

Day	Pain/ Flare Level 👆	Energy ⚡	Stress Level 💭	Water 💧	Healing Foods 🥗	💊	Notes ✏️
Mon							
Tue							
Wed							
Thu							
Fri							
Sat							
Sun							

Listen to your body.

Track your journey. Honor your healing.

How to Use This Table

This 7-Day Healing Wellness Tracker is your invitation to slow down, check in, and gently tune into your body's healing rhythms. There's no right or wrong — just awareness.

Here's how to use each column:

- **Day** – Start with the day of the week or your tracking start date.
- **Pain/Flare Level** – Rate your discomfort from 0 (no pain) to 10 (severe flare). This helps track what foods or habits ease symptoms over time.
- **Energy** – How energized do you feel? Use a 1–10 scale or write "low," "stable," or "high."
- **Stress Level** – Take a moment to reflect on your current stress level. Breathing, prayer, or a walk in nature may shift it.
- **Water** – Track how many glasses (or ounces) of water you drank. Hydration matters!
- **Healing Foods** – List the key healing ingredients you ate that day (like turmeric, leafy greens, sweet potatoes).
- **Supplements** – Note any supportive supplements you took and how they made you feel.
- **Notes** – Anything else? Mood, cravings, sleep, movement, or small victories — write from the heart.

Remember:

This tracker is here to serve you, not stress you. You can use it daily or simply when you feel the need to check in. Healing happens in layers, and this sacred space helps you notice the shifts.

NOTES

"I can do all things through Christ who strengthens me." –
Philippians 4:13

Every day I rise stronger, wiser, and more resilient.

NOTES

"He makes me lie down in green pastures, He leads me beside quiet waters, He restores my soul." – Psalm 23:2-3

Healing is my divine inheritance. I walk forward in grace.

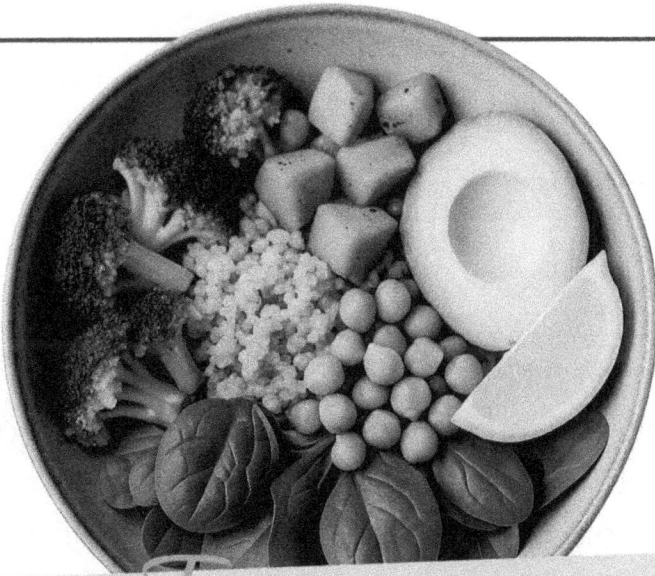

Focus on CHRONIC FATIGUE

"Restoring the Spark Within"

ROOT CAUSES

Chronic fatigue often stems from more than just lack of rest. It can be triggered by:

- **Nutritional deficiencies (especially iron, B12, magnesium)**
- **Blood sugar imbalance**
- **Adrenal fatigue due to chronic stress**
- **Poor sleep quality**
- **Underlying inflammation or immune dysregulation**

For many women, fatigue is both a symptom and a signal — a quiet cry from the body asking for nourishment.

KEY NUTRIENTS

- **Iron** - Supports oxygen delivery
- **B6 and B12** - Boosts energy and nerve function
- **Magnesium** - Relieves fatigue and supports sleep
- **Vitamin C** - Aids in iron absorption and immune resilience
- **Vitamin D** - Regulates mood and immunity
- **CoQ10** - Essential for cellular energy

HEALING FOODS

- **Leafy Greens** - Packed with chlorophyll, iron, and magnesium, leafy greens boost oxygen flow, cleanse the liver, and restore cellular energy.
- **Lentils** - Rich in protein, iron, and B vitamins, lentils support red blood cell production and provide steady, sustained energy.
- **Quinoa** - As a complete protein with magnesium and manganese, quinoa fuels the muscles and stabilizes energy without crashes.

- **Spinach** - Strengthens the blood, nourishes the thyroid, and supports ATP production for deep, lasting vitality.
- **Broccoli** - Broccoli's sulforaphane and vitamin C detoxify the body, balance blood sugar, and protect the mitochondria from fatigue.
- **Pumpkin Seeds** - High in magnesium, zinc, and healthy fats, pumpkin seeds calm the nerves and replenish the body's natural energy stores.
- **Avocados** - nourish the adrenals, balance blood sugar, and provide antioxidants that restore brain and body energy.
- **Lemon** - alkalizes the body, supports the liver, and delivers vitamin C to lift the mood and awaken the spirit.

RECIPES

ENERGIZING QUINOA POWER BOWL

Ingredients:
½ cup cooked quinoa
¼ cup roasted sweet potatoes
A handful of spinach
1 tbsp pumpkin seeds
Olive oil + lemon juice dressing

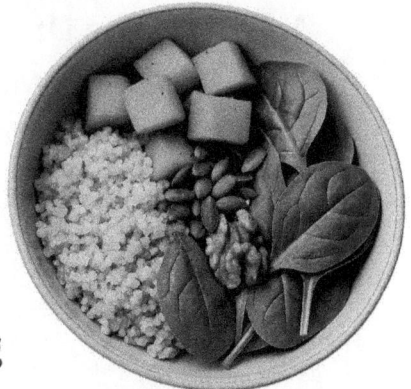

Instructions:

1. Roast the Sweet Potatoes

Preheat your oven to 400°F (200°C).
Cut sweet potatoes into small cubes,
toss lightly with olive oil and spread on a
baking sheet.
Roast for 20–25 minutes, flipping
halfway through, until tender and golden.

2. Prepare the Quinoa

If you haven't already, rinse ½ cup quinoa
under water.
Cook with 1 cup water and a pinch of sea salt:
bring to a boil, cover, then simmer for 15
minutes. Fluff with a fork and let cool slightly.

3. Assemble the Bowl

In a serving bowl, layer the quinoa as your
base.
Add roasted sweet potatoes and a handful of
fresh spinach.
Sprinkle pumpkin seeds on top.

4. Drizzle the Dressing

In a small bowl, whisk together the olive oil
and lemon juice.
Drizzle over the bowl ingredients and toss
gently to coat.

5. Season & Serve

Add a pinch of sea salt and black pepper to taste (optional).

Enjoy warm or chilled for an energizing, nutrient-rich meal.

ADRENAL REBOOT LENTIL SOUP

Ingredients:

½ cup red lentils
¼ cup chopped carrots
¼ cup chopped celery
1 garlic clove, minced

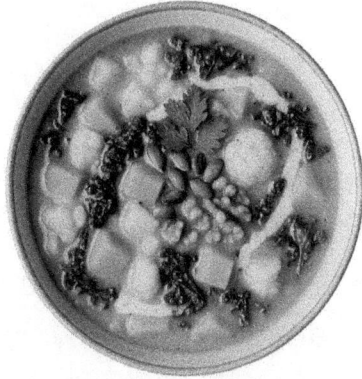

½ tsp turmeric
1 to 2 teaspoons fresh grated ginger
(or 1/2 teaspoon ground ginger if using dried)
2 cups vegetable broth
1 tbsp olive oil
Pinch of sea salt

Instructions:

- Heat olive oil (if included) in a medium pot over medium heat.
- Add aromatics (onions, garlic, ginger) and sauté until fragrant.
- Stir in chopped vegetables and dried spices. Cook 2–3 minutes.

- Pour in broth or water, bring to a boil, then reduce heat.
- Simmer for 15–20 minutes until vegetables are tender and flavors are combined.
- Blend if desired for creamy texture or serve chunky.
- Garnish and enjoy warm as part of your daily healing ritual.

REVIVE & RISE SMOOTHIE

Ingredients:
- 1 frozen banana
- ½ cup blueberries (fresh or frozen – brain + antioxidant power)
- 1 tablespoon chia seeds (fiber + hydration)
- 1 tablespoon almond butter (protein + healthy fat)
- 1 handful spinach (magnesium + iron)
- 1 scoop plant-based vanilla protein powder
- 1 cup unsweetened almond or oat milk
- Optional: ½ tsp maca powder for a natural energy boost
- Ice, if desired

Instructions:
Blend until smooth and creamy. Sip slowly and set an intention for your day.

ENERGIZING ADAPTOGEN TEA

Ingredients:
- 1 tsp dried ashwagandha root
- 1 tsp dried holy basil (tulsi)
- ½ tsp dried licorice root (omit if you have high blood pressure)
- 1 slice fresh ginger
- 2 cups hot water

Instructions:
Steep 10 minutes

Sip daily as part of your healing ritual.

SUPPLEMENT SUGGESTIONS

> **Always consult your healthcare provider before starting new supplements, especially if you're on medications or have a medical condition.**

These gentle, targeted supplements support energy production, replenish nutrient reserves, and alleviate stress on your adrenal and nervous systems. Always consult your healthcare provider before starting any new supplements, especially if you're taking medications.

Magnesium Glycinate
- Supports muscle relaxation, restful sleep, and adrenal recovery.

Vitamin B-Complex (with B12 as methylcobalamin)
- Helps convert food into energy, supports mood, and fights fatigue.

Vitamin D3
- Balances immune function and lifts low energy linked to deficiency.

CoQ10 (Ubiquinol form)
- Powers up mitochondria (your energy factories), especially helpful if you're on statins.

Ashwagandha
- An adaptogen that helps the body cope with stress, fatigue, and anxiety without **overstimulation.**

> Always consult your healthcare provider before starting new supplements, especially if you're on medications or have a medical condition.

L-Carnitine
- Supports fat metabolism and energy at the cellular level, especially helpful for chronic fatigue.

Electrolyte powders (with potassium, magnesium, and sodium)
- Rehydrate and energize, especially if you're low on minerals.

Healing fatigue isn't about revving the engine — it's about refueling the tank.

COACH'S CORNER

Fatigue isn't laziness — it's your body whispering (or sometimes screaming) for deep replenishment. Healing chronic fatigue starts with honoring your body's rhythm and gently returning to balance.

Here are your soul-aligned steps to restore vitality:

- **Balance meals with protein + fiber.** Fueling with the right combo keeps blood sugar stable and energy levels consistent. Think: lentils + greens, quinoa + roasted veggies, or smoothies with chia and protein.
- **Hydrate deeply — beyond water.** Fatigue is often dehydration in disguise. Infuse your water with sea salt + lemon or sip herbal teas like nettle, hibiscus, or ginger to support mineral replenishment.
- **Sleep is sacred.** Establish a nightly ritual — dim lights, read a devotional, or journal your gratitude. Aim to sleep and rise at the same time daily to reset your circadian clock.
- **Step into the sun.** Morning light helps regulate hormones and sleep cycles. Take a 10-minute walk at sunrise or enjoy tea by the window. Nature heals.

- **Magnesium: your nervous system's best friend.** Enjoy magnesium-rich foods like pumpkin seeds, spinach, avocados, and black beans to help calm the body and support restful sleep.

7–Day Healing Wellness Tracker

Day	Pain/ Flare Level	Energy	Stress Level	Water	Healing Foods		Notes
Mon							
Tue							
Wed							
Thu							
Fri							
Sat							
Sun							

Listen to your body.

Track your journey. Honor your healing.

How to Use This Table

This 7-Day Healing Wellness Tracker is your invitation to slow down, check in, and gently tune into your body's healing rhythms. There's no right or wrong — just awareness.

Here's how to use each column:

- **Day** – Start with the day of the week or your tracking start date.
- **Pain/Flare Level** – Rate your discomfort from 0 (no pain) to 10 (severe flare). This helps track what foods or habits ease symptoms over time.
- **Energy** – How energized do you feel? Use a 1–10 scale or write "low," "stable," or "high."
- **Stress Level** – Take a moment to reflect on your current stress level. Breathing, prayer, or a walk in nature may shift it.
- **Water** – Track how many glasses (or ounces) of water you drank. Hydration matters!
- **Healing Foods** – List the key healing ingredients you ate that day (like turmeric, leafy greens, sweet potatoes).
- **Supplements** – Note any supportive supplements you took and how they made you feel.
- **Notes** – Anything else? Mood, cravings, sleep, movement, or small victories — write from the heart.

Remember:

This tracker is here to serve you, not stress you. You can use it daily or simply when you feel the need to check in. Healing happens in layers, and this sacred space helps you notice the shifts.

NOTES

"Come to me, all who are weary and burdened, and I will give you rest." – Matthew 11:28

_____

_____

_____

_____

_____

_____

_____

_____

_____

_____

_____

_____

_____

_____

I honor my body's need for rest, nourishment, and light.

"The Lord is my strength and my shield; my heart trusts in Him, and He helps me." – Psalm 28:7

_____

_____

_____

_____

_____

_____

_____

_____

_____

_____

_____

_____

_____

Energy flows back into my body with every mindful choice I make.

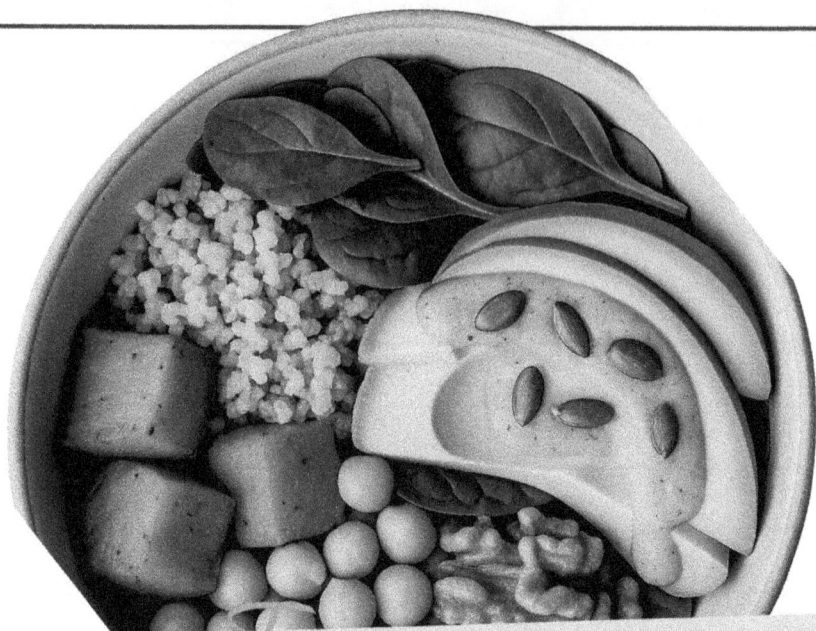

Focus on INFLAMMATION & JOINT SUPPORT

"Easing the Ache, Nourishing the Flow"

ROOT CAUSES

Joint pain and chronic inflammation often go hand in hand. These aches can arise from:

- **Systemic inflammation caused by a poor diet, stress, or autoimmune response**
- **Nutrient depletion (especially omega-3s, magnesium, and antioxidants)**
- **Low physical movement or repetitive stress on joints**

- **Underlying conditions like arthritis, lupus, or fibromyalgia**

Pain may be common, but it is not your destiny. With the right nourishment, you can reduce inflammation and rediscover comfort in movement.

KEY NUTRIENTS

- **Omega-3s** – anti-inflammatory and joint lubricating
- **Magnesium** – reduces stiffness and muscle tension
- **Turmeric (curcumin)** – a powerful anti-inflammatory herb
- **Vitamin D** – supports immune modulation and bone health
- **Antioxidants** – protect joints from oxidative stress

HEALING FOODS

- Chia seeds, flaxseeds, and walnuts for omega-3s
- Turmeric and ginger for inflammation relief
- Leafy greens for magnesium and antioxidants
- Berries (especially blueberries and cherries) for joint protection
- Olive oil and avocado as natural anti-inflammatory fats

RECIPES

ANTI-INFLAMMATORY JOINT SUPPORT BOWL

A deliciously balanced bowl for fighting inflammation and supporting joint health.

Ingredients:
½ cup cooked quinoa
¼ cup roasted sweet potatoes (cubed)
A handful of fresh spinach
¼ cup steamed broccoli
¼ cup roasted chickpeas
¼ avocado, sliced
1 tbsp ground flaxseed or chia seeds
Drizzle of olive oil + a squeeze of lemon juice
Pinch of turmeric and black pepper (optional, for anti-inflammatory boost)

JOINT-SUPPORTING BREAKFAST BOWL

Ingredients:
½ cup cooked steel-cut oats or quinoa
¼ cup blueberries (fresh or frozen)
½ banana, sliced
1 tbsp ground flaxseed
1 tbsp chopped walnuts
½ tsp cinnamon
Drizzle of almond butter or tahini
Splash of unsweetened almond or oat milk

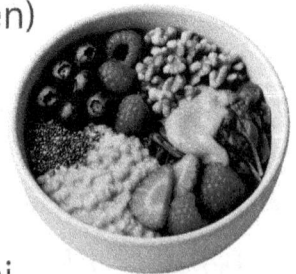

Instructions:

1. Warm the oats/quinoa in a bowl.
2. Top with fruit, flaxseed, walnuts, and cinnamon.
3. Add your drizzle of almond butter and a splash of milk.
4. Mix gently and enjoy this joint-loving, anti-inflammatory breakfast!

ANTI-INFLAMMATORY VEGGIE STIR-FRY WITH GINGER-TURMERIC SAUCE

Ingredients:
For the Stir-Fry:

- 1 tablespoon avocado oil or olive oil
- 1 cup broccoli florets
- 1 small red bell pepper, sliced
- 1 zucchini, sliced
- 1 cup chopped kale or baby spinach
- 1 small red onion, sliced
- 2 cloves garlic, minced
- ½ teaspoon sea salt
- ¼ teaspoon black pepper

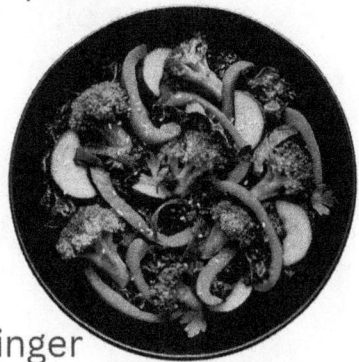

For the Ginger-Turmeric Sauce

- 1 tablespoon fresh grated ginger
- ½ teaspoon ground turmeric (or 1 teaspoon fresh grated turmeric)

- 1 tablespoon tahini or almond butter
- 1 tablespoon coconut aminos or low-sodium tamari
- Juice of ½ lemon
- 1 tablespoon warm water (adjust for desired consistency)

Optional Add-ons:
- ½ cup cooked quinoa or brown rice
- 1 tablespoon hemp seeds or pumpkin seeds on top
- Fresh parsley or cilantro for garnish

Instructions:
1. Prepare the sauce: In a small bowl, whisk together the ginger, turmeric, tahini (or almond butter), coconut aminos, lemon juice, and water until smooth. Set aside.
2. Sauté the veggies: In a large skillet or wok, heat the oil over medium heat. Add the onion and garlic first and cook for 1–2 minutes until fragrant.
3. Add broccoli, bell pepper, and zucchini. Sauté for 4–5 minutes until they begin to soften but still hold color.
4. Stir in the kale or spinach, and sauté for another 1–2 minutes until wilted.

5. Drizzle the Ginger-Turmeric Sauce over the veggies and stir to coat evenly. Cook for an additional 1–2 minutes to warm the sauce.
6. Serve over a scoop of quinoa or brown rice if desired. Top with hemp seeds and fresh herbs for an extra anti-inflammatory boost.

ANTI-INFLAMMATORY TURMERIC GINGER TEA

Ingredients:
2 cups filtered water
1 tsp fresh grated turmeric (or ½ tsp ground turmeric)
1 tsp fresh grated ginger
Juice of ½ lemon
1 tsp raw honey (optional)
A pinch of black pepper (enhances turmeric absorption)

Instructions:
1. In a small saucepan, bring water to a boil.
2. Add turmeric, ginger, and black pepper.
3. Simmer for 10 minutes, covered.
4. Strain into a mug, then stir in lemon juice and honey if using.
5. Sip warm tea to reduce inflammation and soothe joints.

SUPPLEMENT SUGGESTIONS

> **Always consult your healthcare provider before starting new supplements, especially if you're on medications or have a medical condition.**

Turmeric (Curcumin)
- Powerful anti-inflammatory compound that helps reduce joint pain and swelling. Works best when paired with black pepper (piperine) to increase absorption.
- Perfect when stiffness or joint flare-ups are chronic or linked to arthritis.

Omega-3 Fatty Acids (from Algae or Fish Oil)
- These essential fats help reduce inflammation throughout the body and support joint lubrication.
- Great for those with joint stiffness, dry cracking, or systemic inflammation.

Glucosamine & Chondroitin
- These support joint structure and repair by maintaining cartilage integrity and reducing breakdown over time.
- Ideal for aging joints or recovering from injury.

MSM (Methylsulfonylmethane)
- A natural sulfur compound that helps with joint flexibility, pain relief, and inflammation reduction.

- Powerful for rebuilding connective tissue and easing discomfort.

Vitamin D3 + K2

- Supports bone and joint health by enhancing calcium absorption and directing it into the bones rather than joints or soft tissues.
- Best for those with low bone density or indoor lifestyles.

Boswellia Serrata (Indian Frankincense)

- An herbal extract known for its potent anti-inflammatory and analgesic properties.
- Especially useful for chronic joint inflammation or autoimmune-based discomfort.

COACH'S CORNER

1. **Eat a rainbow of anti-inflammatory foods.** Aim for deeply colored fruits and vegetables like berries, spinach, sweet potatoes, and cruciferous greens. These foods are rich in antioxidants that help combat oxidative stress and calm chronic inflammation that contributes to joint stiffness and pain.

2. **Prioritize healthy fats daily.** Include anti-inflammatory fats such as avocado, walnuts, chia seeds, flaxseeds, and olive oil. These nourish cell membranes, cushion joints, and significant for those managing arthritis or chronic joint issues.

3. **Support your gut to support your joints.** An imbalanced gut microbiome can fuel systemic inflammation. Include probiotic-rich foods like kimchi, sauerkraut, or plant-based yogurt, and prebiotic fibers from foods like garlic, onions, and oats to strengthen your digestive defenses.

4. **Stay active with gentle, joint-friendly movement.** Daily low-impact movement—such as walking, swimming, yoga, or tai chi—keeps joints lubricated, supports circulation, and helps reduce stiffness. Even 15 minutes a day can make a meaningful difference in mobility and pain levels.

5. **Get your rest, repair, and sunshine.** Sleep is your body's natural anti-inflammatory time. Prioritize consistent, high-quality sleep and enjoy moderate morning sunlight exposure to help regulate your circadian rhythm and support vitamin D levels, which are crucial for maintaining joint and bone health.

7-Day Healing Wellness Tracker

Day	Pain/ Flare Level ✊	Energy ⚡	Stress Level ☁	Water 💧	Healing Foods 🍲	💊	Notes ✏
Mon							
Tue							
Wed							
Thu							
Fri							
Sat							
Sun							

Listen to your body.

Track your journey. Honor your healing.

How to Use This Table

This 7-Day Healing Wellness Tracker is your invitation to slow down, check in, and gently tune into your body's healing rhythms. There's no right or wrong — just awareness.

Here's how to use each column:

- **Day** – Start with the day of the week or your tracking start date.
- **Pain/Flare Level** – Rate your discomfort from 0 (no pain) to 10 (severe flare). This helps track what foods or habits ease symptoms over time.
- **Energy** – How energized do you feel? Use a 1–10 scale or write "low," "stable," or "high."
- **Stress Level** – Take a moment to reflect on your current stress level. Breathing, prayer, or a walk in nature may shift it.
- **Water** – Track how many glasses (or ounces) of water you drank. Hydration matters!
- **Healing Foods** – List the key healing ingredients you ate that day (like turmeric, leafy greens, sweet potatoes).
- **Supplements** – Note any supportive supplements you took and how they made you feel.
- **Notes** – Anything else? Mood, cravings, sleep, movement, or small victories — write from the heart.

Remember:

This tracker is here to serve you, not stress you. You can use it daily or simply when you feel the need to check in. Healing happens in layers, and this sacred space helps you notice the shifts.

NOTES

"The Lord sustains them on their sickbed and restores them from their bed of illness." – Psalm 41:3

_____

_____

_____

_____

_____

_____

_____

_____

_____

_____

_____

_____

I move with grace and ease as inflammation melts away.

NOTES

"He gives strength to the weary and increases the power of the weak." – Isaiah 40:29

_____

_____

_____

_____

_____

_____

_____

_____

_____

_____

_____

_____

_____

_____

My body is healing. My joints are supported with love and care.

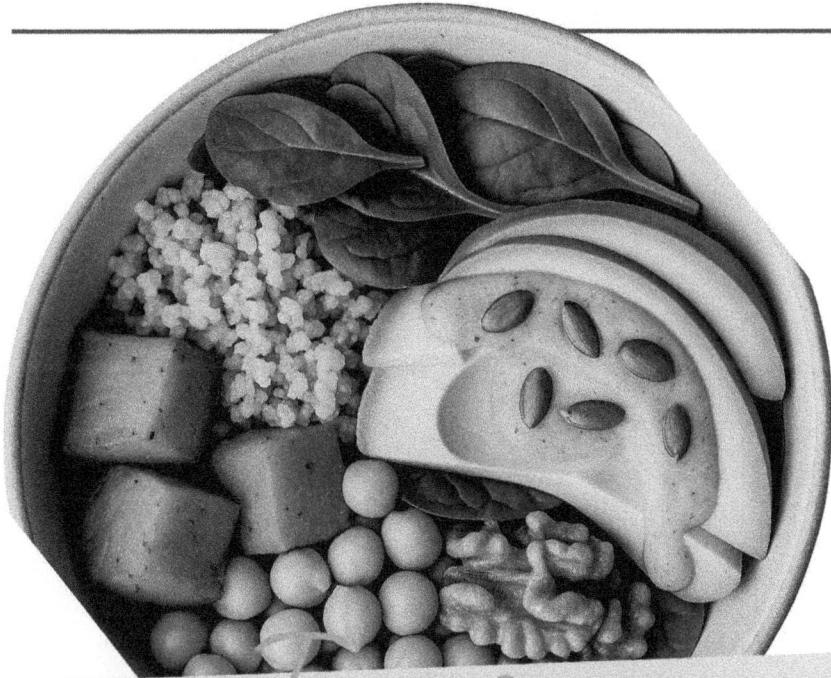

HIGH BLOOD PRESSURE

"Balancing the Flow of Life"

ROOT CAUSES

High blood pressure (hypertension) is often called the "silent killer" because it can go unnoticed while placing serious strain on the heart, brain, and kidneys. Common root causes include:

- Poor diet high in sodium, sugar, and processed fats
- Chronic stress or anxiety
- Obesity or insulin resistance

- Sedentary lifestyle
- Hormonal imbalances or kidney dysfunction

But here's the truth: blood pressure can be influenced positively—often dramatically—through consistent, nourishing changes in what you eat and how you live.

KEY NUTRIENTS

- **Potassium** – helps regulate sodium and relax blood vessels
- **Magnesium** – supports muscle relaxation, including the heart
- **Calcium** – balances vascular tone and nerve signaling
- **Nitrate-rich foods** – improve circulation and vessel flexibility
- **Antioxidants** – reduce oxidative stress that contributes to hypertension

HEALING FOODS

- Leafy greens (like spinach, kale, arugula)
- Beets and beet juice for natural nitrates
- Bananas, avocados, and sweet potatoes for potassium
- Pumpkin seeds, almonds, and black beans for magnesium
- Garlic and hibiscus tea for blood vessel support

HEALING BOWL: THE BLOOD PRESSURE BOWL

Instructions
½ cup quinoa or millet
Steamed kale, roasted beets, sautéed bell peppers
Seasoned black beans or lentils
Avocado slices, pumpkin seeds, and fresh parsley (for toppings)
A drizzle of olive oil and a squeeze of lemon juice

Pair this bowl with a cup of hibiscus tea or warm beet-ginger broth to give your heart a hug from the inside out.

LEAFY GREEN QUINOA BOWL

Ingredients:
- 1 cup cooked quinoa
- 1 cup sautéed kale or spinach
- ¼ avocado, sliced
- 2 tbsp pumpkin seeds
- ¼ cup roasted beets, chopped
- Juice of ½ lemon
- Drizzle of olive oil
- Pinch of sea salt and black pepper

Instructions:
- Layer the quinoa in a bowl.
- Add greens, avocado, beets, and pumpkin seeds.
- Drizzle with olive oil and lemon juice.
- Sprinkle salt and pepper to taste.
- Breathe deep and savor your healing bite.

This bowl is bursting with magnesium, potassium, and fiber—powerful nutrients for lowering blood pressure and nourishing the body gently.

HIBISCUS & CINNAMON TEA

Ingredients:
- 1 tbsp dried hibiscus petals
- ½ tsp Ceylon cinnamon (or a small stick)
- 2 cups hot water
- 1 tsp raw honey or date syrup (optional)
- A squeeze of lemon (optional)

Instructions:
1. Add hibiscus and cinnamon to a teapot or mason jar.
2. Pour hot water over and steep for 10–15 minutes.
3. Strain, sweeten if desired, and enjoy warm or chilled.
4. Sip slowly and let peace flow in.

Hibiscus is known for its gentle blood pressure-lowering properties, while cinnamon supports circulation and insulin sensitivity.

SUPPLEMENT SUGGESTIONS

> **Always consult your healthcare provider before starting new supplements, especially if you're on medications or have a medical condition.**

Magnesium Glycinate or Citrate

- Helps relax blood vessels, reduce stress, and lower blood pressure naturally. This supplement also supports better sleep and nervous system regulation.

Coenzyme Q10 (CoQ10)

- Supports heart function and cellular energy production. Studies show CoQ10 can significantly lower systolic and diastolic blood pressure, especially in those taking blood pressure meds.

Omega-3 Fatty Acids (Plant-Based EPA/DHA)

- Reduces inflammation and supports heart health. Plant-based omega-3s from algae are a wonderful vegan-friendly way to lower blood pressure and reduce triglycerides.

Hibiscus Extract or Tea Capsules

- Acts as a natural ACE inhibitor, similar to some blood pressure meds. Regular use has been shown to gently reduce both systolic and diastolic readings. It's also rich in antioxidants.

SUPPLEMENT SUGGESTIONS CONT'D

Always consult your healthcare provider before starting new supplements, especially if you're on medications or have a medical condition.

Beetroot Powder or Capsules
- Boosts nitric oxide, which helps widen blood vessels.
- This supports smoother blood flow and can help reduce pressure on the heart.

Garlic Extract (Aged Garlic)
- Supports cardiovascular health and helps lower blood pressure.
- Aged garlic has a milder effect on digestion and still provides all the heart-loving benefits, including reduced arterial stiffness.

Potassium (from Food or Natural Supplementation)
- Helps balance sodium levels and ease blood pressure.
- Avocados, sweet potatoes, coconut water, and leafy greens are high in potassium, but a supplement may help if levels are low (under supervision).

COACH'S CORNER

Managing high blood pressure is a sacred act of self-love. Here are five simple, soul-supportive tips to nourish your heart, restore balance, and renew your energy:

1. Sip Smart: Hibiscus & Celery Tea - Herbal allies like hibiscus and celery seed tea can gently lower blood pressure when used consistently. Add a slice of ginger or a splash of lemon, and sip slowly — think of it as self-care in a cup.

2. Season with Purpose - Reduce sodium without sacrificing flavor. Use bold, healing herbs and spices like garlic, turmeric, rosemary, smoked paprika, and lemon zest to create vibrant, heart-happy meals.

3. Breathe to Ease Tension - Inhale peace, exhale pressure. Practice deep, rhythmic breathing for 5–10 minutes daily. Try box breathing: inhale for 4, hold for 4, exhale for 4, hold for 4. This activates your parasympathetic nervous system and supports calm blood flow.

4. Move with Joy, Not Stress - You don't have to hit the gym to benefit from movement. Gentle activities like gardening, walking in nature, dancing while you cook, or stretching while listening to affirmations can help regulate blood pressure and release stuck energy.

5. Hydrate Like It's Sacred - Start your day with a glass of water and continue sipping throughout the day. Staying hydrated helps thin the blood and reduces pressure on your heart. Add cucumber, basil, or mint for an extra touch of freshness.

7-Day Healing Wellness Tracker

Day	Pain/ Flare Level 👆	Energy ⚡	Stress Level ☁	Water 💧	Healing Foods 🍲	💊	Notes ✏
Mon							
Tue							
Wed							
Thu							
Fri							
Sat							
Sun							

Listen to your body.

Track your journey. Honor your healing.

How to Use This Table

This 7-Day Healing Wellness Tracker is your invitation to slow down, check in, and gently tune into your body's healing rhythms. There's no right or wrong — just awareness.

Here's how to use each column:

- **Day** – Start with the day of the week or your tracking start date.
- **Pain/Flare Level** – Rate your discomfort from 0 (no pain) to 10 (severe flare). This helps track what foods or habits ease symptoms over time.
- **Energy** – How energized do you feel? Use a 1–10 scale or write "low," "stable," or "high."
- **Stress Level** – Take a moment to reflect on your current stress level. Breathing, prayer, or a walk in nature may shift it.
- **Water** – Track how many glasses (or ounces) of water you drank. Hydration matters!
- **Healing Foods** – List the key healing ingredients you ate that day (like turmeric, leafy greens, sweet potatoes).
- **Supplements** – Note any supportive supplements you took and how they made you feel.
- **Notes** – Anything else? Mood, cravings, sleep, movement, or small victories — write from the heart.

Remember:

This tracker is here to serve you, not stress you. You can use it daily or simply when you feel the need to check in. Healing happens in layers, and this sacred space helps you notice the shifts.

NOTES

"Peace I leave with you; my peace I give you." – John 14:27

_____

_____

_____

_____

_____

_____

_____

_____

_____

_____

_____

_____

_____

_____

I breathe deeply and release what I cannot control.

NOTES

"A heart at peace gives life to the body." – Proverbs 14:30

_____

_____

_____

_____

_____

_____

_____

_____

_____

_____

_____

_____

_____

_____

With every exhale, I return to calm and wholeness.

_____

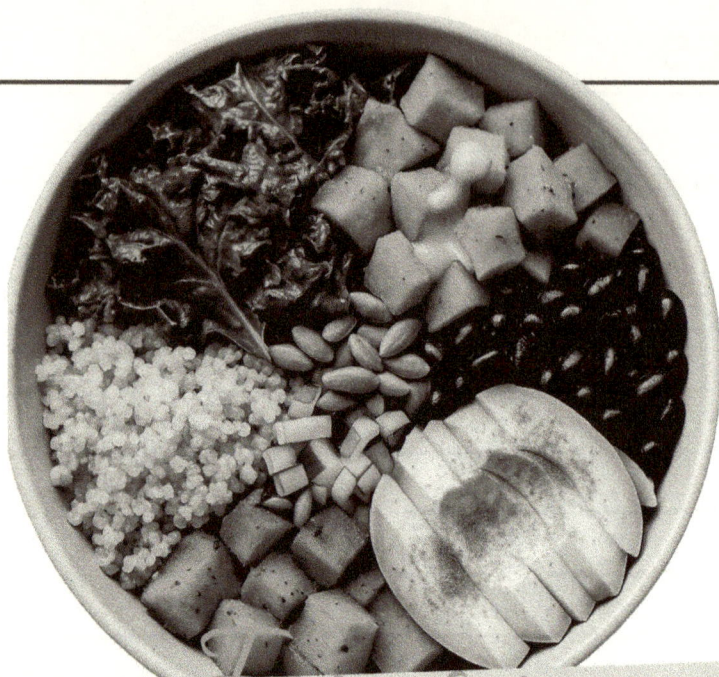

BLOOD SUGAR/ DIABETES

Focus on

"Nourishing Stability, One Bite at a Time"

ROOT CAUSES

When your blood sugar feels like a rollercoaster, your body is asking for balance—not restriction. Healing begins with choosing foods that love your pancreas and support insulin sensitivity. This isn't just about managing diabetes—it's about thriving. Common root causes include:

- Refined Carbohydrates and Sugar Overload
- Chronic Stress and Cortisol Dysregulation

- Inflammation and Oxidative Stress
- Poor Sleep and Irregular Meal Timing
- Sedentary Lifestyle
- Gut Dysbiosis and Digestive Imbalance

KEY NUTRIENTS

These nutrients help improve insulin sensitivity, regulate glucose levels, and reduce inflammation—essential components for maintaining balanced blood sugar:

- **Magnesium** – helps insulin do its job and supports energy.
- **Chromium** – improves insulin sensitivity
- **Fiber** – slows sugar absorption and supports gut health.
- **Cinnamon & Bitter Melon** – natural insulin supporters.
- **B Vitamins** – help metabolize glucose efficiently.
- **Vitamin D3 + D2** - helps modulate insulin secretion and reduce inflammation.
- **Berberine** - a natural plant alkaloid shown to regulate glucose metabolism similarly to metformin.

HEALING FOODS

These foods are gentle on the body, rich in nutrients, and deeply supportive for glucose regulation:

- **Leafy Greens** (spinach, kale, arugula) – Low in carbs and packed with fiber, magnesium, and antioxidants
- **Cruciferous Vegetables** (broccoli, cauliflower, Brussels sprouts) – Support detox and insulin sensitivity
- **Berries** (blueberries, raspberries, blackberries) – High in fiber and antioxidants, with a low glycemic index
- **Chia Seeds & Flaxseeds** – Help regulate blood sugar and improve satiety
- **Avocados** – Rich in healthy fats that help slow the absorption of carbohydrates
- **Cinnamon & Turmeric** – Natural blood sugar regulators and anti-inflammatory agents
- **Legumes** (lentils, black beans, chickpeas) – Rich in fiber and protein, they slow glucose absorption
- **Quinoa & Millet** – Whole grains with more stable glycemic effects than refined carbs

COCONUT VEGGIE HEALING SOUP

Ingredients:

- 1 tbsp coconut oil
- 1 small onion, diced
- 2 cloves garlic, minced
- 1 tbsp fresh ginger, grated
- 1 tsp ground turmeric
- 2 medium carrots, chopped
- 1 small sweet potato, peeled and cubed
- 1 cup chopped broccoli florets
- 1 cup chopped cauliflower florets
- 4 cups low-sodium vegetable broth
- 1 cup unsweetened coconut milk
- Sea salt and black pepper, to taste
- Fresh cilantro or parsley, for garnish (optional)

Instructions:

1. Heat coconut oil in a large pot over medium heat. Sauté the onion, garlic, ginger, and turmeric until fragrant (about 2–3 minutes).
2. Add the carrots, sweet potato, broccoli, and cauliflower. Stir well to coat with the aromatics.
3. Pour in the vegetable broth, bring to a boil, then reduce heat and let simmer until the veggies are tender (about 15–20 minutes).

4. Stir in the coconut milk. Season with salt and pepper to taste.
5. Serve warm, garnished with fresh herbs if desired.

This soup is rich in fiber, anti-inflammatory spices, and healthy fats to stabilize blood sugar while keeping you satisfied.

GREEN GLOW SMOOTHIE

Ingredients:
- 1 cup unsweetened almond milk (or other plant milk)
- 1 small avocado
- 1 handful spinach
- ½ small cucumber, sliced
- 1 tbsp chia seeds or flaxseeds
- Juice of ½ lemon
- ½ green apple (optional, for sweetness)
- Ice cubes

Instructions:
1. Blend all ingredients until smooth and creamy.
2. Taste and adjust with a little extra lemon or apple if desired.

HEALING LENTIL & QUINOA BOWL

Ingredients:
- ½ cup cooked quinoa
- ½ cup cooked lentils
- ½ cup steamed broccoli
- ½ cup roasted zucchini or eggplant
- ¼ avocado, sliced
- 1 tbsp pumpkin seeds
- Drizzle of tahini + lemon juice

Instructions:
1. Arrange quinoa and lentils as the base of your bowl.
2. Add broccoli, roasted veggies, avocado, and pumpkin seeds on top.
3. Drizzle with tahini and a squeeze of lemon before serving.

This bowl layers protein, complex carbs, and healthy fats for balanced glucose response and long-lasting fullness.

CAULIFLOWER STIR-FRY WITH COCONUT AMINOS & SESAME SEEDS

Ingredients:

- 2 cups cauliflower florets
- 1 small zucchini, sliced
- ½ red bell pepper, thinly sliced
- ½ cup chopped bok choy or baby spinach
- 2 tsp avocado oil or coconut oil
- 1 tbsp coconut aminos (a low-sugar soy sauce alternative)
- 1 tsp sesame oil (optional for flavor)
- 1 tbsp sesame seeds
- 1 green onion, thinly sliced
- Sea salt and black pepper, to taste
- Optional: pinch of chili flakes for a bit of heat

Instructions:

1. In a skillet or wok, heat the avocado oil over medium heat.
2. Add cauliflower and stir-fry for 5 minutes until slightly golden.
3. Add zucchini, bell pepper, and bok choy. Stir-fry another 3–4 minutes until tender-crisp.
4. Stir in coconut aminos, sesame oil (if using), and sesame seeds. Toss well.
5. Season with sea salt, black pepper, and optional chili flakes.
6. Remove from heat, garnish with green onion, and serve warm.

Instructions:

1. In a skillet or wok, heat the avocado oil over medium heat.
2. Add cauliflower and stir-fry for 5 minutes until slightly golden.
3. Add zucchini, bell pepper, and bok choy. Stir-fry another 3–4 minutes until tender-crisp.
4. Stir in coconut aminos, sesame oil (if using), and sesame seeds. Toss well.
5. Season with sea salt, black pepper, and optional chili flakes.
6. Remove from heat, garnish with green onion, and serve warm.

Tip:

Pair with a small scoop of quinoa or hemp hearts for added plant protein if desired. This dish is wonderful on its own or served in a wrap or over greens for a light lunch.

BLOOD SUGAR BALANCE BREW

Ingredients:

- 1 tsp Ceylon cinnamon
- 1 tsp dried fenugreek seeds
- 2 slices fresh ginger
- 2 cups hot water

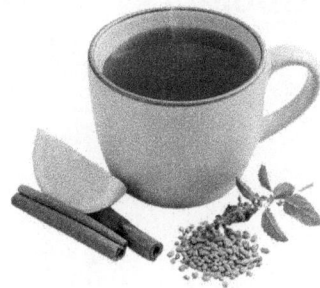

Instructions:

Steep all ingredients for 10–15 minutes. Strain and enjoy before meals to help support blood sugar regulation.

SUPPLEMENT SUGGESTIONS

> Always consult your healthcare provider before starting new supplements, especially if you're on medications or have a medical condition.

Berberine – Helps regulate blood sugar and supports insulin sensitivity.

Chromium Picolinate – Assists insulin efficiency and glucose metabolism.

Ceylon Cinnamon Extract – Naturally reduces post-meal sugar spikes.

Alpha-Lipoic Acid (ALA) – Protects against nerve damage and improves insulin sensitivity.

Magnesium (Glycinate or Citrate) – Essential for blood sugar control and muscle relaxation.

Vitamin D3 + K2 (MK-7) – Supports insulin function and calcium balance (D3 for glucose metabolism, K2 for cardiovascular protection).

Probiotics – A healthy gut improves glucose control and reduces inflammation.

COACH'S CORNER

1. Start Your Day with Protein + Fiber

A breakfast rich in plant-based protein (like tofu, lentils, or seeds) and fiber (like chia, oats, or leafy greens) helps stabilize your blood sugar and energy levels throughout the day. Avoid sugary cereals or white breads — think "slow, steady, and sustaining."

2. Honor the Power of Movement

Gentle movement after meals — like a short walk or light stretching — can significantly reduce post-meal glucose spikes. It doesn't have to be intense. Just move with intention and let your body know you're supporting its flow.

3. Stay Hydrated with Purpose

Sip on herbal teas like cinnamon, ginger, or fenugreek, which may support insulin sensitivity. Avoid sugary drinks and flavored waters. Water infused with herbs, lemon, or cucumber can uplift your body and spirit without the crash.

4. Practice Mindful Carbohydrate Pairing

Don't fear carbs — respect them. Choose whole-food carbs (like sweet potatoes, quinoa, or legumes) and always pair them with fat, fiber, or protein. This combination slows glucose absorption and helps avoid sugar spikes.

5. Create a Peaceful Plate

Eat slowly, breathe between bites, and give gratitude for your food. Mindful eating not only enhances digestion but helps reduce cortisol — a stress hormone that can worsen blood sugar imbalance.

6. Sleep is Sacred

Lack of sleep can increase insulin resistance. Aim for 7–9 hours of quality rest. Set a calming bedtime routine, limit blue light, and wind down with prayer, journaling, or calming music to honor your temple.

7. Track Patterns, Not Perfection

Use a simple journal or tracker to note how you feel after meals, what stabilizes you, and where you need extra support. This empowers you to see progress, not pressure.

7-Day Healing Wellness Tracker

Day	Pain/ Flare Level ✋	Energy ⚡	Stress Level ☁	Water 💧	Healing Foods 🥗	💊	Notes ✏
Mon							
Tue							
Wed							
Thu							
Fri							
Sat							
Sun							

Listen to your body.

Track your journey. Honor your healing.

How to Use This Table

This 7-Day Healing Wellness Tracker is your invitation to slow down, check in, and gently tune into your body's healing rhythms. There's no right or wrong — just awareness.

Here's how to use each column:

- **Day** – Start with the day of the week or your tracking start date.
- **Pain/Flare Level** – Rate your discomfort from 0 (no pain) to 10 (severe flare). This helps track what foods or habits ease symptoms over time.
- **Energy** – How energized do you feel? Use a 1–10 scale or write "low," "stable," or "high."
- **Stress Level** – Take a moment to reflect on your current stress level. Breathing, prayer, or a walk in nature may shift it.
- **Water** – Track how many glasses (or ounces) of water you drank. Hydration matters!
- **Healing Foods** – List the key healing ingredients you ate that day (like turmeric, leafy greens, sweet potatoes).
- **Supplements** – Note any supportive supplements you took and how they made you feel.
- **Notes** – Anything else? Mood, cravings, sleep, movement, or small victories — write from the heart.

Remember:

This tracker is here to serve you, not stress you. You can use it daily or simply when you feel the need to check in. Healing happens in layers, and this sacred space helps you notice the shifts.

NOTES

"Pleasant words are a honeycomb, sweet to the soul and healing to the bones." – Proverbs 16:24

_____

_____

_____

_____

_____

_____

_____

_____

_____

_____

_____

_____

_____

I choose balance, nourishment, and love for my body today.

NOTES

"I will restore you to health and heal your wounds, declares the Lord." – Jeremiah 30:17

_____

_____

_____

_____

_____

_____

_____

_____

_____

_____

_____

_____

_____

My blood sugar is steady, and my life is grounded in peace and purpose.

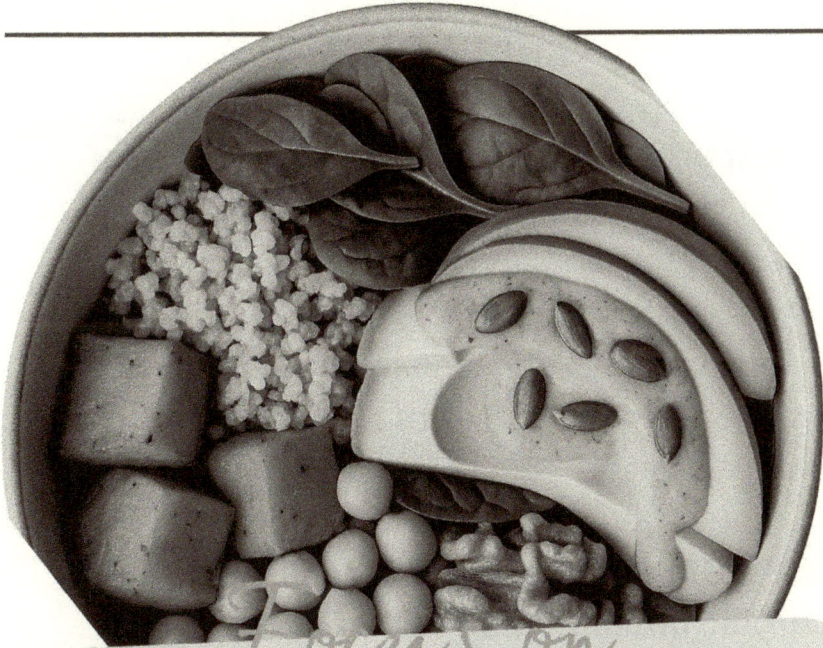

Focus on
AUTOIMMUNE CONDITIONS
"Calming the Fire Within"

When the immune system becomes confused and begins attacking the body it was designed to protect, the result is often an autoimmune condition. Whether it manifests as lupus, rheumatoid arthritis, Hashimoto's, or another diagnosis, the internal struggle can feel both isolating and overwhelming.

But healing is possible.

ROOT CAUSES

You can soothe inflammation, regulate immune response, and nourish your body in ways that invite peace and renewal. This chapter is your gentle starting point for calming the fire within and reclaiming your vitality—one healing choice at a time. Common root causes of autoimmune conditions are:

- **Leaky Gut / Intestinal Permeability**
- **Chronic Inflammation**
- **Nutrient Deficiencies**
- **High Stress and Adrenal Fatigue**
- **Toxic Load**

KEY NUTRIENTS

- **Vitamin D3 + K2** – helps regulate immune activity and lower inflammation
- **Zinc** – supports tissue repair and immune signaling
- **Omega-3 Fatty Acids** – calms systemic inflammation and supports brain and joint health
- **Selenium** – aids thyroid function and detoxification
- **Curcumin** – found in turmeric, reduces inflammatory cytokines
- **Probiotics** – rebuilds gut health and improves immune tolerance

HEALING FOODS

These foods are deeply anti-inflammatory, immune-balancing, and gut-nourishing—ideal for women with autoimmune conditions who want to feel supported and steady in their healing:

- Green & Non-Starchy Vegetables
- Root Vegetables
- Omega-3 Rich Foods
- Bone Broth Substitutes (for plant-based healing)
- Low-Glycemic Fruits
- Healthy Fats
- Anti-Inflammatory Herbs & Spices
- Gluten-Free Ancient Grains (as tolerated)
- Gut-Healing & Fermented Foods
- Liver & Lymph-Supporting Foods

RECIPES

GOLDEN HEALING STEW

A grounding, turmeric-infused veggie stew that calms the gut and warms the soul.

Ingredients:
- 1 tbsp olive oil or avocado oil
- 1 small yellow onion, chopped
- 2 cloves garlic, minced
- 1 tsp fresh ginger, grated

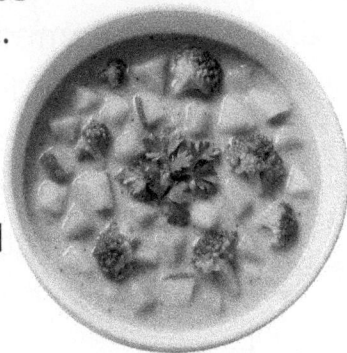

- 1 tsp ground turmeric
- ½ tsp ground cumin
- 2 medium carrots, chopped
- 1 zucchini, chopped
- 1 cup chopped cauliflower florets
- 4 cups low-sodium vegetable broth
- 1 cup coconut milk (unsweetened)
- ½ tsp sea salt
- Juice of ½ lemon
- Fresh parsley for garnish

Instructions:

1. In a pot, heat oil over medium heat. Add onions and sauté until soft.
2. Stir in garlic, ginger, turmeric, and cumin. Cook for 1 minute.
3. Add carrots, zucchini, and cauliflower. Stir well.

AUTOIMMUNE GLOW BOWL

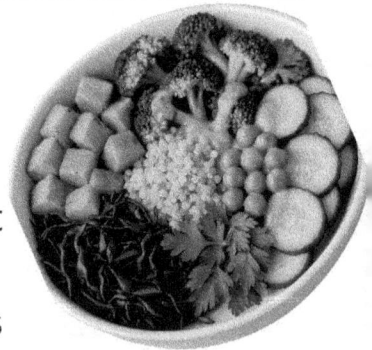

Ingredients:
- ½ cup cooked quinoa or millet
- ½ cup steamed broccoli
- ½ cup roasted sweet potatoes
- ¼ cup sauerkraut or kimchi (optional)
- ¼ avocado, sliced
- 1 tbsp hemp seeds or walnuts
- Drizzle of lemon-tahini dressing (or olive oil + lemon)

Instructions:

1. Layer ingredients into a bowl starting with the grains.
2. Add the warm veggies, sauerkraut (if using), avocado, and seeds.
3. Drizzle with dressing and enjoy warm or room temperature.

Tip: Add a sprinkle of turmeric or cumin to the roasted veggies for extra anti-inflammatory support.

CALM & CLEAR HERBAL TEA

A gentle blend to soothe inflammation and support immune balance.

Ingredients:
- 1 tsp dried chamomile
- 1 tsp dried ginger or a few fresh slices
- ½ tsp turmeric
- 1 tsp dried peppermint or holy basil
- 1 cup hot water
- Optional: ½ tsp coconut oil or splash of non-dairy milk

Instructions:

1. Combine herbs in a tea infuser or jar.
2. Pour hot water over and steep for 8–10 minutes.
3. Add coconut oil or plant milk for a creamier feel.
4. Sip slowly and mindfully.

GOLDEN GUT BOWL
Ingredients:

- ½ cup cooked quinoa
- ½ cup roasted sweet potato, cubed
- ½ cup steamed broccoli
- ½ cup sautéed kale with garlic
- 1 tbsp hemp seeds
- 1 tsp turmeric + pinch black pepper

Instructions:

1. Start with quinoa and sweet potato as the base.
2. Add broccoli and kale.
3. Sprinkle hemp seeds and turmeric + black pepper on top.

Turmeric and black pepper reduce inflammation, while hemp seeds add protein and omega-3s for immune balance.

RAINBOW NOURISH BOWL

Ingredients

- ½ cup brown rice
- ½ cup chickpeas, cooked
- ½ cup roasted zucchini
- ½ cup roasted carrots
- ¼ avocado, sliced
- 2 tbsp sauerkraut
- 1 tsp olive oil + lemon juice

Instructions

1. Place rice and chickpeas in the bowl.
2. Add zucchini and carrots.
3. Top with avocado, sauerkraut, and a drizzle of olive oil + lemon.

Diversity of colors = diversity of antioxidants. This rainbow bowl strengthens the body's defense system and supports gut health.

SUPPLEMENT SUGGESTIONS

> **Always consult your healthcare provider before starting new supplements, especially if you're on medications or have a medical condition.**

1. **Vitamin D3 + K2** - essential for immune modulation and reducing inflammation. Low levels are often seen in autoimmune conditions. Pair with: Healthy fats like avocado or olive oil for better absorption.

2. **Omega-3 Fatty Acids (EPA/DHA)** - help reduce joint pain, support brain function, and calm overactive immune responses. Sources: Algae oil (vegan option), flaxseed oil, or fish oil (if not strictly plant-based).

3. **Turmeric (Curcumin) with Black Pepper** - powerful anti-inflammatory that supports gut and joint health. Look for a supplement with piperine (from black pepper) to enhance absorption.

4. **Probiotics (Multi-Strain)** - a healthy gut equals a more balanced immune system. Probiotics support digestive healing, which is crucial for autoimmune recovery. A broad-spectrum blend with at least 10 billion CFUs.

SUPPLEMENT SUGGESTIONS CONT'D

> Always consult your healthcare provider before starting new supplements, especially if you're on medications or have a medical condition.

5. **L-Glutamine** - supports gut lining repair and intestinal barrier function (a major key in leaky gut-related autoimmune conditions). May also reduce sugar cravings.

6. **Ashwagandha** - an adaptogen that supports immune balance and helps regulate stress hormones, which can worsen autoimmune flare-ups. Not recommended for everyone with autoimmune conditions—always consult first.

7. **Zinc Picolinate** - supports immune function, wound healing, and inflammation control. Take with food to avoid nausea.

COACH'S CORNER

Healing from autoimmune conditions isn't just about eliminating symptoms—it's about nurturing your body back to balance, step by gentle step. These practical tips offer daily support rooted in compassion and science:

1. **Start with Gut Health First**
   Your immune system and gut are deeply intertwined. Begin healing by nourishing your gut with fermented foods (like sauerkraut or coconut yogurt), glutamine-rich foods (like cabbage and spinach), and plenty of fiber. Think of your gut as the garden—tend it, and everything else blooms.
2. **Incorporate Daily Nervous System Calming**
   Autoimmune flare-ups are often triggered or worsened by stress. Use breathwork, prayer, journaling, or gentle yoga to support your nervous system. Even 5–10 minutes of stillness can lower inflammation and re-center your spirit.
3. **Choose Anti-Inflammatory Foods Every Day**
   Eat the rainbow—especially deeply pigmented foods like blueberries, leafy greens, and beets. These foods fight free radicals and support detoxification, helping to calm the immune system and fuel your healing energy.

4. Don't Go It Alone

Autoimmune healing is not meant to be a lonely journey. Lean on your community, reach out for support, and consider a health coach or healing group who understands your journey. Your voice matters—and so does your rest.

5. Honor Your Energy Cycles

Some days you'll feel strong, others tender. That's okay. Learn to listen to your body's wisdom and give yourself permission to slow down when needed. Rest is a form of resilience. You're not falling behind—you're aligning with your healing pace.

7-Day Healing Wellness Tracker

Day	Pain/ Flare Level ☝	Energy ⚡	Stress Level ☁	Water 💧	Healing Foods 🥗	💊 ⃠	Notes ✏
Mon							
Tue							
Wed							
Thu							
Fri							
Sat							
Sun							

Listen to your body.

Track your journey. Honor your healing.

How to Use This Table

This 7-Day Healing Wellness Tracker is your invitation to slow down, check in, and gently tune into your body's healing rhythms. There's no right or wrong — just awareness.

Here's how to use each column:

- **Day** – Start with the day of the week or your tracking start date.
- **Pain/Flare Level** – Rate your discomfort from 0 (no pain) to 10 (severe flare). This helps track what foods or habits ease symptoms over time.
- **Energy** – How energized do you feel? Use a 1–10 scale or write "low," "stable," or "high."
- **Stress Level** – Take a moment to reflect on your current stress level. Breathing, prayer, or a walk in nature may shift it.
- **Water** – Track how many glasses (or ounces) of water you drank. Hydration matters!
- **Healing Foods** – List the key healing ingredients you ate that day (like turmeric, leafy greens, sweet potatoes).
- **Supplements** – Note any supportive supplements you took and how they made you feel.
- **Notes** – Anything else? Mood, cravings, sleep, movement, or small victories — write from the heart.

Remember:

This tracker is here to serve you, not stress you. You can use it daily or simply when you feel the need to check in. Healing happens in layers, and this sacred space helps you notice the shifts

NOTES

"You created my inmost being; You knit me together
in my mother's womb." – Psalm 139:13

_____

_____

_____

_____

_____

_____

_____

_____

_____

_____

_____

_____

_____

_____

My immune system is not my enemy. I am safe and supported.

NOTES

"He heals the brokenhearted and binds up their
wounds." – Psalm 147:3

_____

_____

_____

_____

_____

_____

_____

_____

_____

_____

_____

_____

_____

_____

I am divinely designed to heal, and I trust the wisdom within.

Final Reflections: Grace for the Journey Ahead

Dear Beautiful Sister,

As you close the pages of this book, know that this is not the end—but the beginning of something sacred.

You have taken a powerful step toward honoring your body, nourishing your spirit, and embracing the healing wisdom of the earth. This journey is not about perfection—it's about alignment. Healing is not linear. There will be days of celebration and days of challenge. Through it all, may you hold tight to your purpose and remember that your body is beautifully responsive and capable of repair. You are fearfully and wonderfully made. Psalm 139:14 (KJV).

Let every bite you take be an act of love.

Let every sip be a prayer of restoration.

Let every breath remind you: you are here to live, not just survive.

Whether you are just beginning or deepening your healing path, please give yourself permission to move slowly, rest often, and listen inward.

Your intuition is a compass. Your body is a temple. And your journey is holy ground, but you are not alone. You are surrounded by a circle of wellness warriors, by divine grace, and by the sacred rhythm of renewal.

So, walk forward, beloved—with courage, with hope, and with a heart wide open to possibility.

With all my love,
Patty

About the Author

Patty Johnson Militello
Certified Autoimmune Holistic Nutrition Specialist
| Vegan Transition Coach | Author

Patty Johnson is a passionate guide for women navigating the path of healing from chronic conditions like autoimmune disorders, diabetes, high blood pressure, and more. After witnessing the heartbreaking impact of disease within her own family—and personally experiencing stroke activity, high blood pressure, and diabetes herself—Patty answered a divine call to return to the garden. She believes in the power of food as medicine, faith as fuel, and nature as the original healer.

Through her work as a Certified Autoimmune Holistic Nutrition Specialist and Vegan Transition Coach, Patty has helped countless women reclaim their health through nourishing, plant-powered living. She is the visionary behind Eat the Trees, Drink the Leaves™, a soul-aligned brand rooted in love and well-being.

Patty's mission is to remind every woman that her healing is possible. Her books, workshops, recipes, and journals are all infused with grace, intention, and a joyful invitation to come back home—to the garden, to the earth, and to God.

When she's not writing, coaching, or creating her next nourishing bowl, you can find Patty curled up with a documentary, writing, painting, reading, or spending time with her children in their sacred haven in New Orleans.

📫 Contact Patty
Website: www.eatthetrees.com
Email: support@eatthetrees.com
Facebook: @eatthetrees
Instagram: @eat_the_trees
TikTok: @eatthetrees7

If this book has touched your life or helped you take a step toward healing, Patty would love to hear from you. Your story matters—and sharing it may be the spark someone else needs.

www.ingramcontent.com/pod-product-compliance
Lightning Source LLC
Chambersburg PA
CBHW022340280326
41934CB00006B/714